A B C's
Of
Day Care

A B C's

Of

Day Care

A Caregiver's Guide
with the
Client-Centered
Approach

Margaret Martone

To order additional copies of this book, contact:
Xlibris Corporation
1-888-795-4274
www.Xlibris.com
Orders@Xlibris.com
55743

Give something away every day,
and God will bless you with abundance.

—Margaret Martone

This book is designed to help caregivers present activities to older adults or people with disabilities. The activities are age appropriate for adults with functional impairments.

It is my goal to present activities in a holistic manner and to promote growth or enhance self-image. This book will help you to improve or maintain the functional level of your clients through meaningful activities.

Each activity program should provide ideas for individualized activities, small and large group activities, and the choice to participate or to be a spectator. The activities will meet some of the resident's needs and interests with social, intellectual, cultural, physical, spiritual, and emotional programs.

We will remember the individual differences with each client. The programs should be designed around the client's health status, lifestyle, likes and dislikes considered, abilities and skills by providing opportunities for a variety of types and levels of involvement.

Clients shall be encouraged to take part in activities but may choose not to do so or choose other activities. Remember that a client may choose to just sit and watch others for enjoyment.

Factors to Consider When Planning an Activity

A newspaper reporter will ask the questions who, what, when, where, and why. And those are the questions you should ask too before you plan an activity.

Who are the participants, and who will present the activity? Some people love activities, and some could care less, and this applies to both client and staff.

When an organization finds a crafter, they should develop and encourage every chance they get. Keeping clients busy is healthy. I could write a page on the benefits of well-planned activities.

What type of activity you will present depends on your client population. When dealing with a senior population, remember to keep activities age appropriate. Remember to keep in mind the skill level of your clients. Have the materials ready, and at this point, I would say have a sample. You may need to break a project down into two or more periods. One important thing to remember here is that their finished project may or may not look like yours. If a client gave it their best, then that's the way it is. Please don't fix it to what you like. It isn't your work. Give praise for all and mean it. When we praise, we encourage the participants and others to participate in other activities.

Where the activity will take place is an important factor: lighting (you will need more), space per person (a good rule is to always allow more), sound (will everyone hear the instructions or the speaker?), and temperature in the room. All these factors play a part in the comfort of the client when you present the activity. Other factors to consider depend on the individual client. Know your client and if they have any special needs you may have to consider.

When will the activity happen? Planning the activity should be client centered. What is their day like? Should you plan an activity in the morning, afternoon, or evening? Will this activity happen daily, weekly, or monthly? Try to plan activities when clients are at their peak and not when they are tired, or it's time for a special TV show they love to watch.

Why should you have this activity? Activities should have a purpose. The therapeutic value could be for creative expression to maintain or improve fine motor skills, to recognize religious beliefs or values, to educate, to socialize, to activate the senses, or just to reminisce the past. Activities should be displayed whenever possible. Peer recognition is a great thing.

Planning your activities should show a variety of programs but keep in mind they should have purpose and be centered around the wants and needs of your population.

As the Activities Director

You will develop or improve many skills as you design and present your activities.

You will be organized in the use of your time and resources more efficiently. Being organized will help assistants know their position in the planning and implementing of each scheduled event. It will limit any confusion for clients and staff.

You will become a motivator, dealing with clients and staff. You will inspire them to succeed in their efforts and enjoy a special moment together. You will set the tone for the department.

You will become a goal setter. You will find that you will set a goal for each project, that it has some therapeutic value, and help the client and staff reach their goals as well.

You will develop communication skills. You will improve your verbal and nonverbal ways to communicate to clients and staff. Sometimes, jesters speak louder than words.

You will learn the skills to plan an event and plan too for a backup. You will find yourself planning for "in the event of."

You will become a leader, learning how to get a project started and going through all the steps to the completion. Your manner will not be dictatorial but instructive at all times to both client and staff.

You will promote teamwork—one of the most important skills you have. You will work with the client, staff aides, family, and in some cases, the administration, doctors, or other medical personnel.

The last skill you will develop is your creative skills. As you develop your activities, you will develop some skills or improve skills you have in many areas. Some projects you will enjoy and others maybe dislike.

The important part here is that you develop the program for the client and their interests, that your calendar shows a variety of events and not just what you like. Learning or maintaining these skills will go with you for the rest of your life and will carry over into your personal life. Enjoy the ride!

Planning Together

Make a date to sit down and plan for the month ahead. This planning will allow you to get money or to make reservations. Mark off weekly events like church or shopping. Next, mark off special celebrations, birthdays, or anniversaries and make up some too. I had a happy unbirthday party because we had a month where there were no birthdays to celebrate. At first, the clients thought I was crazy, but everyone sang and enjoyed the cake. They also wanted to know when our next party was. Look for things to celebrate! Next, write community outings and dates for special guests to visit. Plan days to make decorations, write pen pals, and don't forget to mark down the date for the next meeting. How about having a suggestion box? Sometimes, clients have ideas for outings or in-house activities when you are not at work. The suggestion box allows them to write out the idea, and you have another place to get ideas from. Bring the suggestion box to the meeting. You can open it at the start of the meeting, or you can fill in the ideas after the basic needs and wants have been filled in. You should read all suggestions. You should ask coworkers to make suggestions also. We discussed the card catalog, and it is now that you bring it to the meeting. Make new cards or change old ones. Fill in the remaining empty blocks on your calendar with ideas from the catalog.

It will take a lot of time to get a good catalog, but once you do, you'll find that your calendar will have a nice variety. Remember, once you complete your calendar and make a copy for your catalog, it will be a quick reference point next year. Share your ideas with others. You may have a child day care, senior citizen group, or a Sunday schoolteacher who would use the information. I have a friend that has a Cub Scout troop, and I make copies of activities that I think she can use. The connection is good public relations, and they may share some of their ideas they have with you. You should now have a completed calendar—believe me, it gets easier with time. Now the big question, are you going to do everything on the calendar? All I can say here is rarely. There are many outside elements that may cause you to change dates or cancel the activity. Will you have staff, or will they call off? What will you do? Have a backup plan. I live in an area where weather has some effect on going on an outing or not. When roads are bad, you don't go. For people that live in warmer climates or for summer outings, remember to apply sunscreen (apply as needed, and don't forget the top of the ear), wear hats, and sunglasses.

If you have a client on medication, will the person need to stay out of the sun? Should they wear long sleeves? Some clients may be allergic to bug bites. You should find out this information and plan what to do if they should get a bite.

The most important part in planning is that you listen. Some ideas will not work, but you should still give each client time to voice their thoughts. Ask the client what they would like to do if the activity or event planned has to be canceled. If they can't think of anything, you could make some suggestions. The Scout leader tells the troop to be prepared, and that's a good idea for you too.

Therapeutic values: control, anticipation, and patience.

Community Participation

It is very important that we support and encourage community interaction. Belonging to a church group or a service organization can be an experience of joy and of building of self-worth. It gives the client the opportunity to have another circle of friends. You should encourage and support the events they are involved in. See that they have materials or money to attend their meeting or event. If they serve on a committee, see how you can help them reach their goal. Their appearance is an important part of any community event. Are their clothes appropriate for the event? Are their clothes neat and clean? I would encourage a special set of clothes to be worn and set aside for special events. Grooming—hairdo, hair, and nails should be neat and clean.

Will they need any special equipment or transportation?

From the start to the finish, you must be one step ahead of their needs. If a problem should arise, take care of it as quickly and quietly as possible. Hand signals that the client understands can be done quickly with no one knowing. A finger to the lips for quiet time is a lot better than saying, "You need to be quiet and listen now." I was with a group of Scouts and noticed the den mother got everyone to quiet down just by raising her right hand over her head. All the Scouts quieted down and raised their hand for others to follow her cue. It works.

You need to check on your clients' needs while you are out. Do they need to use the restroom? Are they hungry or thirsty? Are they cold or warm? Are they comfortable? Watch for physical signs of needs. Know your client's signals. If John starts tapping his foot, that is a signal he needs to use a restroom. Check your client's special needs too. If they wear glasses, are they cleaned daily or as needed? If they have a hearing aid, are the batteries in it working?

I know all this may sound overwhelming at first, but after a while, you will do a head-to-toe survey in a few seconds. You will anticipate the wants and needs as you get to know your client better. You will take courses to help you in an emergency and how to deal with them each day in a professional manner.

Outside Resources

Be creative about recruiting and using volunteers. Here is a list to get you started in planning your calendar of events and for getting speakers:

- Your local chamber of commerce
- The library
- Local churches and religious organizations
- A community calendar
- Fair association (Check for calendar of events.)
- The yellow pages of the telephone book
- Local craft stores (See if they have instruction classes.)
- Newspapers
- Hospitals for speakers
- Zoos
- Movie theaters
- Restaurants
- Animal shelters for pet therapy
- Amusement parks
- Museums
- Sport centers
- Radio / TV station

Make a list of nonprofit organizations for events and speakers:

- American Legion
- Rotary
- Boy Scouts
- Girl Scouts
- Veterans or VFW
- Lions Club
- Masons
- Fire companies
- Center for Performing Arts
- Stadiums, arenas, and athletic fields
- Women's and men's groups
- Senior centers and school events

Now that I have you thinking, I'll bet you can come up with another list. Remember to plan around what the client likes and their physical needs.

With regard to outings, please do your homework. Look for specials, discounts, amenities, times, directions and try and get to know a contact person. Plan for the client's safety and comfort as well. Events should not cause stress but some enjoyment. Take some extra clothes, water, medication, phone list for emergencies and a cell phone, pen, and paper. Here too you may want to design a checklist. I have listed a few things to consider, but you will need to design your list around your client. If you are working for a company, check to see if they have a list.

Community Information Assessment

Name of activity:_____

Contact person: _____

Address/directions: _____

_____

_____

_____

Telephone number: _____

Cost per person: _____

Ratio of staff to clients:_____

Discounts: _____

Amenities:_____

Parking: _____

Hours open:_____

Days closed: _____

Wheelchair or walker friendly: _____

Others:_____

_____

_____

_____

_____

Would you attend this activity again?_____

Are there any safety issues? _____

What changes would you make?

_____

_____

_____

What would you take during the outing? _____

_____

Gathering Information

Card catalog your information. You can save yourself a lot of time by forming an index file of activities—one section on outings and the other on the arts and crafts. You can network with others by sharing this information.

For community card:

Name of activity (and contact person):
Address (directions on how to get there):
Telephone number:
Discounts:
Amenities:
Hours open:
Wheelchair or walker friendly:
Others:

After a visit, update your card with remarks and whether you would do the activity again or what changes you would make to make the outing more enjoyable for you and your client. Don't forget safety issues.

Activities and crafts card (who, what, when, where, and why)

List activity:
Materials needed:
Staffing:
Cost:
Therapeutic values:
Changes from past experiences:
Length of time for activity: (If more than one hour, you may want to break the activity into segments or break for a drink or small snack.)
Where will the activity take place?

It is important that you have the client participate in forming these cards. Would they like to do the activity again? How often would they want to do the activity? In the planning of the activities, what changes would they like? The more information they give you will help you better plan the next activity.

Activities and Crafts Assessment (Who, What, When, Where, and Why)

Name of activity:_____

Date of activity:_____

Materials needed: _____
_____
_____
_____
_____

Ratio of staff/clients:_____

Cost: _____

Therapeutic values: _____

Changes from past experiences: _____
_____

Length of time for activity: _____

Snacks to be served: _____

Where will the activity be held? _____

Would you do this activity again?_____

How often should you present this activity?_____ `

Staff comments: _____
_____
_____
_____

Client comments: _____
_____
_____
_____

Creating an Activity

For each activity you plan, you will find a group of steps, and knowing the steps will better organize your time and money.

1. What is the concept or basic idea? As a coordinator, you will be on the lookout for ideas daily. After a while, your coworkers and clients will come to you with ideas and know you as the person who will carry them out.

2. What modifications will you make to present this activity to your clients? Will you have to do some prep work before you bring it to the table?

3. You will have to gather materials. You should always use materials you have and rotate your stock when adding to your supply cabinet.

4. Make a sample. When you are making a sample, you will become aware if this activity will work with your current population. During the making of the sample, you will again find that you will make modifications to the plan.

5. Bring the activity to the table. Evaluate who will need help and how much help you should offer. Encourage independence or teamwork. Make suggestions only when necessary.

6. Praise during and after the project and be specific. "I just love the red color you used in the painting of the rose." The bits of encouragement will make the client feel they are doing a good job. Don't be judgmental or say negative remarks. This is what they feel and want to do.

7. Display works of art whenever possible. If a client does not want to display the project, that's okay too. If they just want to take it to their room or home, well, again this is their choice.

8. Clean up after the project is completed. Ask each person to clean up their own area and put the materials away. Make a note if you are running out of anything or if you need to replace an item.

9. Should you update your activity card? Do you want to do this activity again? Make some notes if you have time.

10. Complete your documentation. If the client will be taking the project home, be sure the completed activity is placed in a bag or folder for travel and not just shoved in a pocket.

Client Assessment

Name of client: _____

Wants	Needs	Hobbies
1.	1.	1.
2.	2.	2.
3.	3.	3.
4.	4.	4.
5.	5.	5.

Likes	Dislikes	Crafts
1.	1.	1.
2.	2.	2.
3.	3.	3.
4.	4.	4.
5.	5.	5.

Skills or limitations:

____Uses a scissor
____Can print/write
____Follow simple directions
____Can use paints
____Can draw
____Use paper punches
____Use stapler
____Help set up
____Help clean up
____Seeks attention
____Exhibits good behavior
____Exhibits poor behavior
____Exhibits good manners
____Works well with others
____Works best alone
____Likes animals
____Likes TV
____Demonstrates difficulty
   in communicating

____Limited time on task
____Enjoys outings
____Completes projects
____Needs help in the following:
1.
2.
3.
4.
5.
____Handles own money
____Possesses good hygiene
____Needs assistance with hygiene
____Demonstrates good table manners
____One-on-one in public
____Physical assistance
____Fear of pets
____Demonstrates good verbal skills
____Understands gestures

Safety Behind the Wheel

If you have more than two people in the car/van, you can easily be distracted. Have some travel rules and remember that the radio is a distraction. The volume should not be so high that you will not hear if a client has an emergency, or that you will not hear an emergency vehicle.

Check clients' seat belts each time you get in the vehicle. If traveling with a group, do a head count before you leave and after each stop.

Know your clients' special needs for traveling and if they will get carsick on a long trip. Have an emergency car kit. Check with AAA for updated *Driving Survival and Emergency Car Care Guide* books. They also have kits that you can buy for under $100. Let's face the fact you may well be the first responder at the accident. Have a cell phone. Have an emergency photo card for each client. If you have an accident and can't communicate, these would be valuable to emergency personnel. Emergency cards should be updated whenever there is a change in information. Check them once a month anyway. Have the cards in a plastic bag and mark the bag Emergency Information in large letters on both sides. Place the emergency information bag in a side pocket of the driver's door or the best place visible, depending on your vehicle.

Know your client's special needs and plan ahead. Will you need a wheelchair? Clients may not use a wheelchair but they may enjoy and see more if they had one. I had a client who only used a wheelchair at the fair. She would never be able to cover all the events without it. Her comfort and safety was my main concern.

Learn and use good body mechanics when lifting a wheelchair in and out of your vehicle. The last thing you want to do is pull a muscle.

When traveling with a group, remember to take what you can handle. If a person has special needs, you may want to consider one-on-one or take clients that can be more independent with you.

Make up a list of things you might need in an emergency. I carry water and cups, a fire extinguisher, rubber-and-cotton work gloves, a small set of tools, a tarp, and a first aid box.

All facilities have fire evacuation plans, but few are trained in the event of an accident. You should be proactive and discuss what clients should do in the event of an accident. You could make this a learning activity.

Safety starts by being prepared.

Travel Assessment

Name of company: _____

Mailing address: _____

Emergency telephone number: _____

Insurance company: _____

Vehicle check:
    Driver's license _____
    Tires and spare _____
    Oil _____
    Full gas tank (mileage noted) _____
    Fire extinguisher_____
    Road map_____
    Written directions _____
    Emergency photo cards_____
    Tickets or boarding passes _____
    Adjusted mirrors _____
    Seat belts_____
    First aid kit_____
    Pencil and paper _____
    Emergency sign or cones _____
    Flares_____
    Tools and jumper cables _____
    Gallons of water and cups_____
    Tarp_____
    Gloves: latex and work _____
    Medications_____
    Luggage_____
    Throwaway camera _____

Comments _____
_____
_____
_____
_____

Materials

For a start-up program, let's start simple and buy materials as you better understand your client's skills and needs. You should have a cabinet or designated area to keep your supplies. Depending on your clients, you may need to keep a lock on it for safety reasons. I have found that marking the shelf with designated areas for paper products, games, and crafts are very helpful. A place for everything and everything in its place will save you time, money, and help other staff find items to do activities as well.

- VCR player
- Happy ending / funny tapes
- Cassette / radio player
- Cassette tapes (music they enjoy)
- A good exercise tape (to maintain or improve range of motion for their age and physical condition)
- Parachute (for a group exercise. Play some music during this exercise too.)
- Bean bags (for range of motion and hand-eye coordination)
- A large ball for a group or one-on-one activity
- Construction paper (seasonal colors to start or an assortment package)
- Paint (seven basic colors)
- Paintbrushes in assorted sizes
- Glue and glue gun with sticks
- Scissors (right- and left-handed)
- Needles (for stringing beads, and a small box to keep them in)
- Beads
- Crayons (seven basic colors)
- White drawing paper
- Card stock and envelope
- Nail care products
- Bingo game
- Dominoes

- Checkers
- Two deck cards
- Throwaway camera
- Stickers
- Computer
- Garden supplies

Once you complete your client assessment, you may find that you should add other interests to the list.

Remember to keep an inventory and to replace any broken items. Remind everyone to rewind tapes after use and report broken equipment and take suggestions for new tapes.

Clients may choose to bring their own materials to an activity. A client may choose to work on one pet project while others do the planned activity. Remember this is a program for the client's free time. So much of their day is planned for them, and showing independence of choice should be encouraged. This is a time for you to praise them and show your support. Check and see that they have everything they will need. Give help when they request it.

The Interview

How can you plan an activity when you don't know the person? Well, you can. And it is a general calendar, and if that's what you want, it's okay. But if your heart is in your work, you won't be happy with that! You'll want a calendar that will show you care and love your work. When my father was in a nursing home, I checked out the activity calendar, and I saw a general stereotypical activity calendar. Now, let's see what we can do.

First, get to know your clients. Sit down one-on-one and ask them about themselves. What do they like to do? Do they have any hobbies? Can they share the hobby with others? Get to know their beliefs and values, wants, and needs and make a list of each. I would do an update each year as the list might change from time to time. If a form is not available, make up your own. Plan around their wants and the available resources you have.

The Budget

When it comes to the budget, you may have to be a scrooge, penny-pinching miser. You will become a master at recycling and caring for your materials. When I was working, people used to come to me with packing materials, plastics, and more and say, "What can we do with this?" Thank God! I have a mind that starts clicking, and usually, I would come up with a project or two in about five minutes. But that's me and my MacGyver mind. My point here is, if you are that quick thinker, that's a plus; and if not, well, find one. You must know someone who can make a rose out of a coffee filter (yes, you can).

Anything you can recycle will save your budget. One time, we had a Hawaiian theme, and we made a Tiki hut on our kitchen counter. What did we make the grass hut out of? Brown paper bags. We cut the bottom out of the bag (save, paint, and cut out large leaf). Then we cut the bag open, laid it flat on the table, and painted it green. When the bags dried, we cut strips, one-half inch wide, through three-fourths of the bags. We overlapped and taped together the bags just like they would if they were putting together a grass roof. We then painted coffee filters with pink, yellow, and purple and made them into flowers. We added some other decorations and had a luau. You need to use your resources wisely, and recycling is a great way to do that.

For that project, the staff brought in the shopping bags. The coffee filters came from our kitchen, tape, from office supplies, and the cost to the activities budget was a few pennies for the paint. As you work on activities, you will change the way you look at everything. At one point, I found myself almost like being in a game, on a hunt for free stuff. And let me say, this can become an addiction. You guessed it; I liked my job. Here too if you like your job, it will show in your work, and you will find it hard to work with people who don't. So don't take it personally. You are there for the client. How you present yourself is your connection, and it will show in your work. No one says a job has to be work. Why not enjoy what you are doing? You're going to be at it a long time.

Things to Remember

Time Management

Organizing the presentation. You are the focal point, and it is up to you to teach through activities. Walk around as you speak and note who is listening. Look at the client's face, and note if you see a puzzled look. Maybe you're not getting through. Your posture, tone, and expression are all part of presenting an activity.

Offer examples and encourage creativity. Be sensitive to the limitations of each client. It doesn't have to be perfect. Remember to check the client's physical condition. Is the client tired? Remember, some of the clients get up early and put in hours before the activity. They may be on medications, which can make them sleepy. Have a finished product to show your clients.
Sometimes, telling someone with a disability isn't enough; but if you have a finished product, you may help them understand what you are saying.

Every effort deserves praise. It is important to set a time for your activity. If the activities' purpose is to relax the client, then don't stress them out. How long an activity should be depends on the client and the activity itself. Any activity over one hour should have a break. When doing an activity, remember other factors. Do they have enough light? Do they need help? Are they warm enough? Do they need to be toileted? Are they trusty or hungry? Who is sitting next to them? How much space do they need? How much time on task can they do? You must be constantly watching and know the warning signs for a change or when to stop the activity.

Equipment and Budget

This is a tough area because most budgets I have seen are bad. When the going gets tough, get it for free.

Making something out of recycled materials will become a game, and it is one I just love to play. Anytime I pick up something to toss in the trash, I think, *How can I use this?* You would be surprised as to what you can make. Thrift is another word I love. Taking one thousand place mats at a cost of about $15 (or maybe a local bank would offer you a box) can become place mat art, with stickers, markers, magazine cutouts, and photocopies of the client's family. Oh my, I could make so many projects.

Recycled cardboard from the supermarket is another throwaway product you can make use of. Can you get colored paper? I don't mind asking another department for anything. I have used shredded paper (to line an Easter basket), cotton balls, and Q-tips, and when the maintenance department is around, I scavenge around and get copper tubing (wind chimes), scraps of wood, and so much more. Sometimes, people will tell me, "I have something I think you could use," and I'll look at whatever it is. And nine out of ten times, I can make something out of it.

Sample Projects and Pretesting

It is important to be thinking of each client when making a sample—what they will be able to do and whether they will they need help. Put yourself in their shoes for a few minutes. After you iron out all the bugs, you should have a finished project to show them. When they complete the activity, remember to praise them for all the hard work. If you can put it on display, then be sure you do even if it is only for the day. It isn't going to look like yours, but it is their best, and that's wonderful!

Residents' Rights
Residents have rights. Remember, if they do not wish to participate, that is their choice.

Community
Residents should be encouraged to participate in community events. They should be encouraged to join community organizations as well. Contact local groups and ask if someone would sponsor your client.

Attitude
I am talking about yours. The way you present yourself is so important. You need enthusiasm and passion. If you hate your work, the client will pick up on that, and they will not get excited to participate. The way you walk and stand are nonverbal cues that people can pick up

on. What you say is important, and how you say it reflects even more. You are there to make that hour enjoyable for them. The bottom line is that this is your job!

Cultural Awareness

You need to know many things in presenting activities, and cultural awareness is an important aspect. All I can say here is that you need to keep learning as much about your clients as you can. What do they believe in? Each person will be different. Everything from religious beliefs, politics, music, and even one's personal beliefs will play a part in who that person is. This is a tough area but use it to celebrate them and make others aware of who they are. Make everyone's holiday your holiday too . . . party, party!

Keeping Track of Cleanliness

Keeping your hands clean is important, and you need to wash them often. Make sure you are having your clients wash their hands too, and if they can't wash them, then you help and wash them for themselves.

The work area should be cleaned after each activity, meal, or snack.

Food as an Activity

Almost everyone will participate in this activity. We must again look at the client. What kind of diet are they on? Are there foods they should avoid? Will I have to cut it into bite-size pieces? Will I have to change how it is served? Foods should appeal to the senses. It should taste, smell, feel, and look enjoyable. This may take a little time, but it is time well spent with a picky eater. Portion control is important also. If a client cannot measure a proper amount, then have premeasured portions or serve the client the proper amount. Try to make the food served something that everyone can have. We should not put ourselves in a position where we have to tell a client they cannot have a food. It will not hurt everyone to eat sugar-free cookies or Jell-O.

Individual Plan and Modifications

Each client will have an individual plan. Knowing each plan is an important part of your job and getting to know your client's likes and dislikes, wants, and needs will play an important part in how you serve them. Keep a keen eye slightly ahead of them. Know what is important to them. Watch for the unsaid cues that tip you off, and know how to react to what you see. Physical changes could signal you to a bigger problem.

Range of Motion

Know the range of motion of each clients—hands, arms, and legs. Don't ask a client to extend beyond what is comfortable. You do not want a client to feel pain. You should not push them because this could cause an injury. If a client says it hurts, then stop.

Verbal and Nonverbal Communication

Use words that the client can understand and never talk in another language. Your tone for the words reflects meaning. Are you loud or soft-spoken? How would you feel? Your unspoken image says more than you think. How you walk, dress, talk, and present yourself say more about you and your interaction with the client. Believe me when I say clients will learn to read you like a book, and they will pick up when you are in a good mood or not. Try to make each day the best you can.

Location and Space

Location and space available is important, as well as the number of people in that space. Remember to allow extra space. No one likes to be stuffed in like sardines in a can. When you pick a location, remember the lighting, temperature of the room, sound system, and seating.

Documentation

If it is your duty to complete documentation, you should cover some main facts. First, you should list the name of the activity and whether the client was able to follow procedures or if they needed help. What was the time on task? Did they just hurry through it, or did they work meticulously, covering every task? Did they use materials as they were intended, or did you see a misuse? You should also point out the therapeutic value for the event and say whether they enjoyed the experience or not. The last part would be, did they complete the project or not?

Exercise for January

Below is a list of activities for thirty-one days. In this exercise, you should have a blank calendar. Place events that are personal to your client or group—birthdays, anniversaries, Founder's Day (if you work or an organization), and any other personal events. Remember to celebrate everything, and you can even make up some crazy events. Now review the national holiday list and add them to your calendar. Would you like to add a flower of the month? Cutouts or stickers could be placed around the calendar for color and interest. You could add a color theme as well; let's say that everything will be black and white for January. For my last suggestion, pick a theme and run with it. Build your calendar around it and get everyone thinking of ideas for the calendar. Ours for this exercise is "It's for the Birds." The monthly celebrations for January are National Soup Month, Hot Tea Month, and Eye Care Month just to name a few.

Letter writing. In the first week, we will see pen pals because it is the Universal Letter Writing Week. You can call this event Letters and Cards, Send a Note, With this Pen, or *L* is for Letter. Try to make the calendar interesting, and if it is an activity you plan to have monthly, change the title. You may be doing the same activity, but just change how you present it.

Finger painting. This is one of the activities that you can do yourself. Mix one envelope of unflavored gelatin, two and one-fourth cups water, one-half cup cornstarch, and three tablespoons of sugar. That is your base, and now you can add a flavor for some aromatherapy. Divide into containers and add two or three drops of food coloring to each container. Be sure you put down some newspaper or a plastic tablecloth before you start because this can be one messy activity.

The two activities listed above may cost just pennies from your budget, but if you can get items donated or can get supplies from the office or the kitchen, well, you know me by now—cheap, cheap, cheap.

Attracting birds (review activity plan) and stringing beads. Feeding the birds and watching them at the feeder is a great January activity. Clients will enjoy making some treats, and this activity can also vary if you plan to run it a few months. Our fine-feathered friends at the feeder, well, you can see what I mean.

Stringing beads was one event that my clients really enjoyed. I didn't mind spending money for this activity. The craft stores have a vast variety for you to pick from, and in some of the stores like AC Moore, they show finished products, and this should give you more ideas. I would stress here to take care of your supplies. If they come in a bag, you should find a small container to keep them in. An open bag of beads is no fun to be picked up, and I should know. I really like this activity because it is creative, promotes fine hand-eye coordination, and your clients have a finished product to enjoy. When the activity is over, remember to give praise to everyone.

Papier-mâché. Papier-mâché is another messy activity. You will need a supply of torn newspapers and mixture of flour and water, which will be your paste. This is another activity that is budget friendly. Your activity will need drying time. I found it best to let the product dry a day or two. What are you going to make? That depends on you and your clients. Our first project was a fruit bowl. For this activity, you will take a large bowl and cover it with clear wrap. Then lay strips of newspaper covered with paste over the outside of the bowl. You should have at least three layers of paper, allowing a drying time between each completed layer. When the bowl has dried completely, apply a coat of white paint, let it dry again completely. You could apply cutout pictures of fruit to the outside or draw some pictures and paint appropriately. For the last step, you will need to apply a clear coat of acrylic paint.

Beanbag toss. For this activity, you could buy a beanbag toss game or make your own. If you wish to make the beanbags, you will need four-inch squares of material (at least ten pieces), a small plastic bag for each beanbag, a needle, and thread (or a sewing machine). You can decorate a plain tablecloth with your targets painted on it, and the last thing you need is, of course, beans. For our activity, we placed one cup of beans in a small plastic bag. We sewed close three sides of the material and inserted the bag of beans. We then closed the last side, and our bag was complete. We painted circles using a dinner plate for our pattern. When the painted circles dried, we placed numbers in each circle for points.

Tissue-art snowman decoration. You will need three circles of different sizes cut from sturdy cardboard. The size of the snowman depends on several factors. What will it be used for? How many clients will be working on the project? Will the project take a few days to complete? For our project, we made a life-size door decoration. We cut three-inch squares of white tissue paper, crimpled the paper into small balls, and placed the paper balls in a box the first day. Oh, you should know we had six clients working on this project. The second day, I divided the six clients into groups of two, gave them one of the cardboard circles, glue, and the crimpled pieces of tissue paper. Each group pasted the tissue balls on the cardboard circle until the cardboard was completely covered. When they completed that, we made facial features cut from construction paper and glued them over the tissue balls in the appropriate places. We added a hat, scarf, and some black circles to represent buttons, and we joined the three circles to complete our snowman. We placed him on the front door for the month. This project took three days to complete, cost pennies, and most importantly, it had value. Everyone that visited our unit made a comment about our snowman; we even gave him a name—Jack.

Armchair travel. You can pick up a video at your local library or check with a travel agent in your area. Pick a country to travel and learn about in the comfort of your own place. One of our trips was to Germany, and while the clients watched the video, I heated up some of those large pretzels. By the time the video was over, the aroma had wafted to the dayroom, and everyone enjoyed a special snack as we discussed the film.

Exercise. It is now a proven fact that exercise is beneficial to our bodies. If possible, you should incorporate exercise into a daily routine—a thirty-minute walk, some stretching to improve or maintain range of motion, or lifting of weights. The type of exercise will depend on your client. There are tapes available, and here is where I wouldn't mind spending some money. A good tape will last a long time, and you should remember to rewind the tape when you are finished.

Horticulture in January, why not? Check at your local Agway or garden center for some winter activities. I called my state extension office, and they sent me instructions for planting paperwhites. We also started some baby spider plants given to us by a good-hearted staff. You can root them in water two or three weeks before your planting date.

Bingo here too. I would invest in a good game. Our clients enjoyed this event so much that I put in on our calendar as a weekly event. Bingo prizes can be purchased at the dollar store or be asked at a staff meeting for unwanted item that can be used for bingo prizes. Some of the best items—stationeries, hair-care products, hygiene supplies, jewelry, hats, and socks.

Scrapbook designing. A page in a scrapbook is a great activity. You can use stickers, cutouts from cards or magazines, pictures from activities, old-road maps, ribbons—well, the list is endless.

Hobbies. If a client has a hobby, I would suggest you learn something about it too. Can you incorporate what they know into an activity for others? This is a great learning project for you and other clients. I once had a client that collected patches. You know, the ones you sew on shirts or jackets. Well, he had them in a shoe box and brought them to the table for show-and-tell one day. It seems that over the past ten or fifteen years, this man collected patches wherever he went, and if he saw a patch on someone, he would ask them how he might get one. Most people said they would send him one for free. He had a great collection. When I got home, I checked my wood supplies and found a piece of four-by-four paneling. I then called a friend who was a carpenter and asked him if he would cut some molding for a frame around the paneling. I brought all the pieces to work and offered a one-on-one project for building a display board for his patches. Other clients watched as we put the display board together and glued the patches on the board. My client enjoyed the attention and peer recognition as he told the story behind each patch. Each house member was then on the lookout for patches to give him. This project cost nothing to my budget but was very therapeutic for everyone.

Photo magic. Through the years, I have made it a point to take photos of my clients to incorporate into activities. One of my last activities was to take pictures of clients dressed up for Halloween, and I brought my photocopier to work so that each client could watch their picture develop. The pictures were placed in a cutout card for them to give to their family for Halloween. A few pennies for a great communications activity.

Watercolor art. For this project, you may want to place some newspaper on the table. You will need watercolor paper, a tray of paints, and a small cup of water. I used the plastic medication cups for my individual water cups. It holds a small amount of water, and if it should spill, well, it is easier to clean up. You should encourage each client to pencil draw a picture to be painted. For this project, we drew pictures of birds because our theme for the month was "Our Fine-Feathered Friends." Your painting will need time to dry.

Making musical instruments. For this project, we made a drum using decorated oatmeal containers (which we painted and decorated in another activity session). We cut plastic bags one inch larger than the open end of the container and secured it in place with a heavy rubber band. We put a tape in the tape player and played our drums to the beat. We also sang along just for fun.

Message in a Bottle. If you want to see a good movie with your clients, well get this one staring Kevin Costner. Make some popcorn and keep your tissue box handy. After seeing this movie I thought we could make an activity with this concept. We bought pint and quart canning glass jars and as our color for the month of February will be red and white, we painted the lids red, and the bands white. We needed materials to put in the jar so we got some sand and a few pretty shells and stones to put around the base of our picture. We put the sand in the jar, them positioned the picture; we placed the stones and shells in next. You can use twigs, nuts, or anything else that will help you stand up your picture. We next decorated the outside of the jar with raffia tied in a bow, and for a little added charm we hot glued a few tiny shells on the lid. Don forget to put in a message on the back of the picture. You will be the hit of the day on valentines with this one of a kind gift.

Rhythm band. Making musical instruments out of recycled materials can be lots of fun. You could put some beans in a plastic Easter egg and glue it shut, make a drum out of an oatmeal container, or make a rain stick. For the rain stick, you will need a paper towel tube, card stock, glue, foil and rice or pebbles. Trace the end of the tube on a piece of card stock; now draw another line half an inch wider than the open end of the tube. Cut the disk out and cut around the disk half an inch from the edge. You should put the cuts about one-fourth inch apart. You will need two of these. Place some glue around the bottom of the tube and bend the card-stock disk in place. You will need to let this dry. Cut a piece of foil about eighteen inches wide. Now crumple it widthwise. It should be about as long as your tube. Place half a cup of rice (or pebbles) in the tube and glue the last card-stock disk on the end. Let it dry completely and decorate your rain stick with paint, stickers, or paper.

Beads. Make a batch of dough by mixing two cups of flour, one cup of salt, and enough water to make a dough. Make into small balls and then push a toothpick through to make the hole and bake for one hour at three hundred degrees. Remove from the oven and paint from your favorite color. After your paint has dried, string your baked bead with thread or dental floss.

Black paper art. You will need a piece of black construction paper and a piece of white chalk. Discuss things you could draw with the chalk, keeping with the black-and-white color theme. A snowman or penguins are just two things that are black and white that you may consider.

Dominos. Have a contest to find the best domino player. If you have these chips in your odds-and-ends box, you can use them to make a pin. Take a chip and paint a snowman on the blank side, let your work dry, and then glue a pin back on the other side. Let glue dry completely, and you have a one-of-a-kind work of art to wear.

Book review. Have your client pick a book that is age appropriate. Set up a time when it is quiet, read a chapter, and have a discussion about what you have read. Take turns reading, and if your client cannot read, then read the story to them. Discuss key points and give each client a chance to speak.

Nail care. Keeping your clients' (both male and female) nails clean is just a part of good grooming. You should check nails daily for breakage or foreign matter. You can set aside a time to soak the fingertips, trim the nails, and paint them too for an activity. Don't forget to rub on some hand lotion when you are finished.

Dancing to the music. This is an activity you could present once a month. Each month, you could learn a new dance and write the type of dance you will be doing on your calendar. Let's see—"Let's Twist Again," "Tennessee Waltz," "Let's Boogie"—well, you can think of a catchy title too.

Photo-frame art. Keeping with our color theme, our frame will be black and white. For this project, I bought a five-by-seven wooden frame at AC Moore. We then painted the frame white. We let the paint dry and then painted black dots around the frame. You could also add black-and-white buttons, dice, or poker chips just to be creative.

Animal shelter. Contact your local shelter and ask them for a wants-and-needs list. Review the list with your clients and pick out one or two ways you can help. This could be a monthly activity—changing the class plan to meet the shelters' needs, shredding newspaper for bedding, collecting blankets and cutting them to size, or making puppy treats are not only fun, but you are providing a community service.

Board games. Our theme colors continue into our board game too. For this project, we are going to make our own checkerboard game. Glue a piece of poster paper on to a piece of cardboard. Draw lines for each square and have the clients color in the black ones with marker. Let the board dry. For the board pieces, paint a set of milk carton lids black and another set white. When you finish playing the game, store the tops in a plastic bag.

Memory box. Years ago, cigar boxes were used by children to keep their treasures. Today, you can buy a wooden box and decorate it for a project. Your client will have a unique box with their personal touch. We cut out magazine pictures and lined the inside of the box. We then applied a few coats of clear acrylic paint. We painted the outside and gave it time to dry. Here too you could paint their name or glue on ornaments of choice.

Road safety. Being safe in the car is just part of the job. Present a miniclass on the wearing of your seat belts and why it is important. Check with your local police department and see if a member could put on a program and offer to go to the police station for the program. If it is arranged, don't forget the follow-up activity of making a thank-you card.

His name was Martin. The third Monday in January is set aside to celebrate the birthday of Martin Luther King. Review his speech "I have a dream."

Cinnamon hearts. We don't eat them! This is a project to hang in your home. Mix equal parts of apple sauce and cinnamon to form a type of dough. Roll out one-half inch thick and cut with a two-inch heart-shaped cookie cutter. Poke a hole in the top center of the heart, about one-half inch from the edge. This hole is for the ribbon you will need to hang the heart. Let it dry a few days on a cookie sheet lined with a paper towel. These are great to give next month on Valentine's Day, so make a few for giving too.

It's in the soup. January is National Soup Month, so why not make it an activity too? Have the soup of the day be your client's choice. With a few ingredients like celery, carrot, onion, meat, and broth, you have an activity that arouses the senses of touch, smell, and taste.

No bake candy. For peanut butter crunches, cream together one cup of peanut butter, one cup confectioners' sugar, and two tablespoons of milk. Shape teaspoon-sized portions into small balls and roll in chocolate rice crispies. Melt one package of chocolate morsels in the microwave or double boiler. Now, dip each ball into the melted chocolate and place on wax paper. When you have completed your tray, chill till the chocolate has set. Place in a plastic container and store in the refrigerator.

Tea tasting. Gather some special teas with different flavors: mint, orange, Earl Grey—your choice. Four or five different types should be enough. Read the packages for the company's description of the tea. For the tasting, I used small plastic medication cups. They hold about thirty cubic centimeters, just enough for a taste. We talked about the color, taste, and where the tea was grown. When we finished our discussion, each person was served their favorite with a few cookies.

Exercise tape. If you don't have a tape, just form your own exercise routine. Design it around your client's physical condition, and don't forget to check with nursing for special needs. Walking in the park is physical exercise, and if the weather is bad, don't forget a mall walk. Senior citizens are walking there all the time because it also provides a social group to interact with.

Show-and-tell. This activity is not just for children. Encourage your client to show pictures of their family or a hobby they enjoy. Ask questions of interest like where the pictures were taken, or, if a hobby, how long have they've been doing it. Use open-ended questions to encourage conversation.

Bingo.

Alphabet soup pin. Take a box of alphabet pasta and look for letters to form words. Glue the letters in order on a two-inch piece of card stock. Glue a pin back on the other side, and you have a great pin. You could make an It's My Birthday or Marty Loves Ann pin and save it for a special day.

Community lunch. Everyone enjoys going out for lunch. Enjoy the experience by adding a search game on your way to the restaurant. The first person to see a gas station gets Hershey's Kisses, or the first person to see an animal gets a gumdrop. You will keep your clients busy and alert.

Board games. Client's choice. Remember to keep the game clean and put away all the pieces when the game is over.

Fire prevention. Fire Prevention Week is in October, but fire safety is a daily and year-round practice. When you design your activity, be sure your facts are correct. For this activity, I invited a fireman to come and talk to the clients about using an oxygen mask. Each client was told to listen to the fireman and to follow his directions. We gave the fireman a thank-you card, and he joined us for lunch.

Suggestion box art. For this activity, you will need a shoe box. Cover the lid and bottom of the box with white paper. Now, be creative and let your client decorate the box. Encourage clients to put ideas for crafts, outings, or other events written on paper with their name in the box.

Singing to the oldies. When I was growing up in the fifties, we had a blend of artists who were so unique that even though they are gone, their music is still enjoyed today. Floyd Cramer, Johnny Cash, Burl Ives, Elvis, and even Ol' Blue Eyes himself, Frank Sinatra, were just a few. Some of the music during my mother's days were still being heard. So ask your clients who they would like to listen to and go ahead sing and dance. Remember, these are their favorites, not yours.

Gift tags and bags. It is a lot easier to put a gift in a bag than to try and wrap it sometimes. You can buy plain gift bags at the $1 store, and with some bits and pieces, make them not only works of art but great conversation pieces. For this project, we will do a birthday bag. You will need a plain brown bag, some cutouts from old birthday cards, and some markers. Repeatedly write Happy Birthday all over the bag. Now, from old birthday cards you have saved in your recycle box, cut out the front panel from a birthday card and glue it to the front of the bag. Take another front panel from a card, fold it in half, punch a hold in the upper left corner, insert a ribbon or yarn, and you have a tag to tie on the bag.

Community service project. For this project, we visited a nursing home and brought magazines we have collected from all the staff. Be sure the magazines are complete and not cut up. Roll the magazine and tie a ribbon around it. Place them in a basket for easy passing. Try and have a variety, and don't forget magazines men enjoy like sports car or wrestling. You may want to read a few stories from *Good Old Days* or an article from *Better Homes and Gardens*. It is a time to share not only the magazine, but a piece of you too.

Show and tell. Pick a topic like show-and-tell family photo time and give the client time to talk about a photo they have. It could be a family, friend, or even a pet. Encourage a brief statement about the photo and where it was taken. If the client has a hard time expressing their thought, ask open-ended questions and give them time to think.

Church supper. It is important that your clients have community interaction as often as they can. You don't have to be a member if it is a fund-raising event. Just be sure that your client is dressed for the event and practices good table manners. Portion control should be based on their diet. Food allergies and hypersensitive reactions to foods should be noted. Cut foods that are too large, and if the client is a possible choker, keep them next to you and monitor closely.

Can you kazoo? This is a musical instrument that almost everyone can play. It is a lot of fun to make music and to exercise your lungs as well. Each client should have their own kazoo, and they should be washed with soap and water before you put them away.

Scouts to visit. Interaction with children may well correlate with another group and their goals. The Scouts visit can be a community service project for them and an activity for you. Your visit should end with a simple treat. Our Scouts came and made dream catchers with our folks, and we served milk and cookies.

Decorate cupcakes. Taking part in a meal preparation could be setting the table, pouring the water, or decorating cupcakes for supper. The clients iced the cupcakes and then put different types of sprinkles and candies on top. It was a lot of fun, and I heard some boasting as they were passed around.

Bingo.

Auto safety. The first step in safety is being prepared. If you work for a company and they have a transportation department, well, check with them to see if they have a written plan. And if not, how about making up one? Our instruction for today was how to use a seat belt. If your client is unable to buckle up independently, then you must do that for them each time they get in your vehicle. Show them how to use a seat belt and then have them try it independently. You should know who will need your help with this because it's the law.

Sponge painting. This basic skill can be used to make place mat art, or for our project, we made wrapping paper. We cut two sponges into the shape of stars. We dipped one sponge in red acrylic paint and dabbed it on our plain white paper. We then took the other sponge and dipped it into blue acrylic paint. We took a piece of card stock and made a small matching card to go with the paper.

Banner art. This is one of the best activities to do. You should have a piece of white paper—twenty-four inches wide and five feet long. Looking ahead, Valentine's Day is just around the corner so make a Valentine's banner—Happy Valentine's Day! It could be the lettering with drawings of hearts of all different sizes around the completed words. Color in the letters and hearts. What you could write in the hearts are couple's names or copy some of the cute sayings on those heart-shape candies. Why not pass a few of those around when you are working on it?

Current events. Keeping up with events in the world around us is just part of living on this planet. Keep in mind topics that your client enjoys reading about. It could be sports, politics, or just Dear Abby for fun. You will need a newspaper or a magazine to draw your discussion from.

Flower arranging. For this activity, well to be honest, I got my flowers from our local undertaker. Sometimes, there are so many flowers given when someone passes, and they don't know what to do with them. I was looking to recycle all the time and asked my friendly undertaker to consider my clients, and we got some of the nicest baskets you ever wanted to see. Don't forget that baskets and ribbons can be used in other projects too. You should also check at your local garden center for odds and ends.

Activity meeting. Now is the time to have a meeting to plan for next month. Gather up your cards for February, select a theme, pick your colors, open your suggestion box, and get all your clients involved in the planning. You will need a few days to get your materials together.

Folklore. Pick a folklore character and design a program around them. We picked Paul Bunyan for this activity. I found a book about folklore at our library, and a friend drew a picture of Babe the Blue Ox for us to color. We had a discussion about folklore and how they get started.

Community breakfast. If you are budget minded, this is the meal to eat out. We have a local restaurant that is more than just a business because they go out of their way to make eating out a great experience for my clients. They will come out and sing a round of "Happy Birthday," and if we spill something, it is no big deal. They have heart and know we are all just a heartbeat away from a disability too. Thanks, Spanky!

Explorer I, the first U.S. satellite launched. This is the anniversary of the launching of our first satellite. You could discuss space exploration and follow the history of events from Kitty Hawk to the Kennedy Space Center.

Well, you have just had a brief trip through the January activities calendar with some personal thoughts and information. Try and keep in mind the client-centered approach, budget, staff, and time when planning next month. Gather your team players and delegate, delegate, delegate. Don't take on more than you can handle; we don't want staff burnout.

SUN	MON	TUE	WED	THU	FRI	SAT
1 Rem Pals Finger paint shirt Decorations (Seasonal)	2 attracting Birds String Beads	3 paper mâché Bean Bag Toss	4 Tissue Art Video Arm Chair Travel	5 Exercise Horticulture	6 Bingo ScrapBooking	7 Hobbies Photo magic
8 Water color Art Making Musical instruments	9 paper basket Take Decoration Rhythm Band	10 Baking Beads carols (your choice)	11 Black paper art Dominoes	12 Reading Book review Mail Call	13 Bingo Dancing to the music	14 Photo Frame Art Ornament Shower
15 Board game Memory Blg	16 Instruction Road Safety most in Bathroom Stationery Art (Rule-on transition)	17 Cinnamon Hearts Oil on the Soup	18 No Bake Candy Tea Tasting	19 Exercise type Show + Tell photos & family	20 Bingo Alphabet Soup Nature Song time	21 Community Lunch Board Games
22 Five Presentation Suggestion Box Art	23 Singing to the oldies Making gift Bags + Tags	24 Community Service project String Tell	25 Church Supper Can you Kazoo	26 Scouts to Visit make cookies Decorate Cup Cakes	27 Bingo Auto Safety Drive	28 Sponge Painting Banana Art
29 Current Events Flower Arranging	30 Activity meeting Folklore Paul Bunyan	31 Community Breakfast Explorer I 1st US Satellite			Bingo	

A Year of Celebration

Below, you will find a list of reasons to celebrate. This is only a partial list of events to help you complete your calendar. This is a great time to study our values, differences, and celebrate diversity. I will give you six ideas for each month, but you can make up your own too. I will also give you the flower of the month and the gem of the month. You may incorporate them into your theme for the month or as a monthly decorating idea.

January. When old man winter blows in the cold, you may find yourself in the house more than you would like. Planning table activities and events that play on the senses can fill in the time. Creating something from the kitchen combines math skill, hand-eye coordination, and don't forget the effects of aromatherapy. This could be a perfect time to set and work on some goals too.

Flower of the month is the carnation, and the gem is the garnet.

1 : New Year's Day. Set some goals for the week, month, and year.
4 : Trivia Day. Go around the table passing out trivia. "Did you know that . . . ?" "It is a fact that . . ."
8 : Elvis's birthday. Play music and sing some of his best songs.
18 : Maintenance Day. If you have a maintenance department, have a luncheon for them.
19 : Martin Luther King's birthday. Read "I have a dream."
20 : Inauguration Day. Read about past presidents or watch the inauguration on TV.

February. This is the month for presidents and love.
Flower of the month is the primrose, and the gem is the amethyst.

12 : Lincoln's birthday. Read the history of one of our greatest presidents.
14 : Valentine's Day. Make and send cards.
16 : President's Day. Discuss what it must be like to live in the white house.
22 : Washington's birthday. Make up a game . . . e.g., How many Georges do you know?

15 : Ash Wednesday. Discuss the Christian belief and symbols of faith.

29 : Leap year. Discuss the calendar, and why we have an extra day every four years.

March. This month we celebrate St. Patrick's Day; March wind
Flower of the month is the daffodil, and the gem is the aquamarine.

6 : Remember the Alamo. Discuss the American heroes that fought at the Alamo

8 : Daylight Saving Time begins. Spring ahead or fall back.

8 : International Women's Day. Discuss the differences between men and women.

10 : Harriet Tubman Day. A great woman in history. Review her life history.

12 : Girl Scout's Day. Invite a local troop for a joint activity.

17 : St. Patrick's Day. Have a party, sing Irish music and dance.

April. Showers bring May flowers/Easter
Flower of the month is the daisy, and the gem is the diamond.

1 : April Fools Day. What is a jester?

5 : Palm Sunday. Discuss the holy day in the Christian faith.

9 : Passover. What does Passover mean to the Jewish client? How is it celebrated?

10 : Good Friday. A time of reflection.

12 : Easter Sunday. Easter egg hunt. Special phone calls

22 : Secretaries Day. Remember to say thank you. A token gift from the heart.

May. Do you remember the Maypole?
Flower of the month is the lily of the valley, and the gem is the emerald.

5 : Cinco de Mayo celebration. Discuss independence in Mexico.

6 : Florence Nightingale. History. The lady with the lamp.

8 : V-E Day. The end of World War II.

10 : Mother's Day. I remember Mama. Tell a story about your mother.

16 : Armed Forces Day. Discuss the different branches of the military.

25 : Memorial Day. What does it mean when I say "I pledge allegiance"?

June. A time for planting and walks in the park.
The flower of the month is the rose, and the gem is the pearl.

1 : Children's Day. Encourage interaction with babies and small children.
4 : National Frozen Yogurt Day. Have a yogurt-tasting party.
6 : Pet Appreciation Week. Donate puppy bones and visit the nearest shelter.
8 : Best Friends Day. Write a letter to your best friend or visit a friend.
14 : Flag Day. Discuss the American flags design. Create a personal flag.
21 : Father's Day. I called him Father, Dad, Pop, and Daddy. What's in a name?

July. Red, white, and blue, picnics, marching music
The flower of the month is the water lily, and the gem is the ruby.

4 : Independence Day. Celebrate with a barbeque.
9 : Park and recreation celebration should be as often as weather will allow.
12 : Parents' Day. Study your family heritage. Where were your parents born?
16 : Ice cream. Make a sundae or a banana split.
23 : National Hot Dog Day. Enjoy hot dogs on the grill.
39 : Comedy Celebration Day. Show a movie or video.

August. Sports . . . walks . . . fresh air.
The flower of the month is the poppy, and the gem is the sardonyx.

2 : Friendship Day. Write a letter to a friend or have them over for lunch.
5 : National Mustard Day. Taste test three or four different types of mustard.
7 : International Clown Week. Face painting . . . dress up like a clown.
19 : National Aviation Day. Have lunch at a small airport.
20 : Homeless Animal Day. Visit a shelter, donate dog/cat food.

September. Back to school, apples, and seasonal change.
The flower of the month is the aster, and the gem is the sapphire.

2 : VJ Day
7 : Labor Day. If I could only be (name a profession), I could . . .
11 : Patriots Day. What makes a patriot (name one)?

19 : Rosh Hashanah. Why did the Jewish people want to leave Egypt?
21 : International Day of Peace. Design a peace poster.
28 : Yom Kippur. Make and serve some Jewish food.

October. Falling leaves, harvest time, a cornucopia of food and color.
The flower of the month is the calendula, and the gem is the opal.

12 : Columbus Day. Find Spain on the map; find the route to the New World.
16 : Bosses' Day. Celebrate by taking your boss out for lunch.
16 : Dictionary Day. Have a spelling bee.
26 : International Red Cross Day. Host a CPR class.
31 : National Magic Day. Read the story of Harry Houdini.
31 : Halloween. Decorate, dress up, and have a party.

November. Turkey, stuffing, pie, and thanksgiving.
The flower of the month is the chrysanthemum, and the gem is the topaz.

1 : Daylight Saving Time Ends. Nocturnal animals.
3 : National Sandwich Day. Who was the Earl of Sandwich?
3 : Election Day. Vote and review the ballot.
11 : Veteran's Day. Attend a community observance. Check with a VFW Post.
26 : Thanksgiving. Say a special prayer.
27 : Black Friday. Don't shop. Address your Christmas cards.

December. Christmas shopping, wrapping gifts, singing, and decorating.
The flower of the month is the holly plant, and the gem is the turquoise.

7 : Pearl Harbor Day. Invite a veteran to lunch.
12 : Hanukkah. Celebrate with music and a special food.
21 : First day of winter. Make snowflakes.
25 : Christmas. Celebrate with family and friends. Open gifts.
26 : First day of Kwanzaa. Celebrate African heritage.
31 : New Year's Eve. Make party decorations and celebrate.

Documentation

Documentation is always an important part of your activities program. At time we search for words to express our program or event. Below is a list of words to help you.

Therapeutic value creative, social, long term and short-term memory, self-esteem, reminiscence, education, communication skills, faith, exercise, or sensory stimulation.

Aroma stimulation . . . using fragrances in a activity.
Communication skills . . . listening, and patients in waiting your turn.
Creative expression . . . maintains or improves talents.
Cultural enrichment . . . development, artistic, social or religious.
Decision making . . . alternative choices, or preferences.
Enjoyment . . . satisfaction, amusement, entertainment, or hobby.
Educational . . . intellectual, scholastic, or academic.
Empowerment . . . permits. enable, and make a choice.
Flexibility . . . changeable, able to adjust to change.
Hand & Eve Coordination . . . able to move hands and eyes, synchronized.
Independent Functioning . . . without direction, self governing.
Long Term Memory memory of the past.
Light Exercise . . . with-in ones physical endurance, or range of motion.
Large Group Activity . . . congregation, club, party, meeting.
Mental Stimulation . . . emotional enjoyment, pleasure.
Motor Skills . . . maintain motion, movement, range.
Motivation and adjustment . . . . Ability to change.
Nurturing . . . , gentle, tender.
Reminiscing . . . to remember or recall.
Relaxation . . . rest, vacation.
Recycling . . . use again, to help the environment
Short Term Memory . . . In the present, reality.
Spectator Participation . . . to watch, or listen.
Small Group . . . Three to six people.
Self-Esteem . . . respect, confidence, assurance.
Socialization . . . Participation
Structured . . . arrange, conceive, conceptualize.
Sensory Awareness . . . mind, reason, opinion, understanding.
Self Reliance . . . Depending on ones skill, Independent or others.

Painting Rocks

If you live near a river, well, the store is open. You have an endless supply and use for river rocks. Very small ones can be decorated. Apply a magnet to the back, and you have a refrigerator magnet.

Decorate larger ones for doorstops and even larger ones for garden art projects. For this project, we will make a refrigerator magnet. The weight of the rock will determine the size of the magnet. Look for flat thin stones, about the size of a matchbook. At your local craft store, buy round flat magnets, good strong glue, acrylic paint, and paintbrushes. Take a large trash can bag, cut off the bottom, and cut up the side. This will form a tablecloth, which can be rolled up and tossed in the trash after the project is completed. Paint each rock, let dry, and glue magnet to the back. You may decorate the front with gems, cutouts from magazines, and well, you get the picture. If you use cutouts of paper, you may want to cover with a clear acrylic paint to maintain paper color.

Therapeutic values: creative expression, good decision making, and a purposeful project.

Suggestion Box

For this activity, you will need a shoe box and paper to wrap the top and bottom portion of the box. You should cut a hole in the top just big enough to slide a piece of paper through. I cut a four-by-one inch thick hole in the center of the box. You will wrap each part separately because you have to open it each month to review the suggestions. You can decorate the box and should write Suggestion on the side. You should place the box where all clients have access to it. We had ours in the dayroom, on the coffee table. When a client comes to you during the month with ideas, tell them to write it down and put them in the box. If your client can't write, take a minute and write it for them. Take a few minutes before the meeting to review the suggestions. Sometimes, notes are not clear, and it will give you time to review the suggestion with the client rather than at the meeting.

Recycle time! I used a road map to cover our box.

Educational

Don't forget that an activity can be educational too. Whether you get out the atlas and discuss Iran or draw a picture of the heart and discuss the flow of blood, it is important that your facts are correct, so check them online or at the public library when planning the activity. My clients and I would gather each morning and read about the weather and discuss how it will affect our day. We would also have a laugh when the weatherman was wrong. Then we would read an article and discuss what was important. Looking at the story, we discussed who, what, when, where, and why. Remember to keep the topic moving and encourage everyone's input. The activity should take about one hour. If your activity is longer, break for a beverage or snack. When working with a group, you may find a client who gives too much information. If this happens, try to incorporate the roundtable approach where each person takes a turn and then you move on to the next. I used this approach because at times, I would have clients with too much information and clients who never gave input. I would help the quiet client by asking an open-ended question and encourage them with prompts and praises. When you find a client that disrupts the group, give them something else to do away from the group or maybe with another staff. It is just as important that they be kept busy, maybe more so.

You could incorporate company or nursing department goals. Start with basic skills such as daily living skills, and then once they are mastered to the best of their ability, move on to fun things. Sometimes, you may want to spend a few minutes just to refresh the skills learned. It doesn't hurt—you know you have fire training every year for a reason.

Pinwheels

Read all the instructions for this activity before you start. Materials for this project: an eight-inch square piece of card stock, scissors, a small nail or pin, markers, a pencil, and a twelve-inch stick to attach the pinwheel to. This basic design can be made in any size you want. The only rule is you need to start with a square piece of paper. Place a ruler diagonally from corner to corner, a draw a line. Do the same with remaining corners. You should have an X through your work.

Now is the time to decorate both sides of the paper. To form the individual section, you will cut from the edge three-fourths of the way toward the center on each line. Now take the right top corner and fold toward the center, take left top corner fold toward the center, overlapping the first piece, take the bottom left corner and fold toward the center, overlapping the other two pieces. Now take the lower right corner and turn toward the center. Place a pin into the middle and secure all four points to the center. Place a small bead on the pin; this will allow a space between the paper and the stick. You will need a hammer to tap the point of the pin into the stick. Try not to drive the pin through the stick because you will have a sharp pin sticking out. In the event you do, tap the point over and cover with a piece of Scotch tape. No sharp points sticking out, please. The wheel itself can be used to make a wreath or to substitute for a bow. I needed a bow for a birthday gift, so I cut a piece of card stock and randomly wrote Happy Birthday, Mike all over the card. Then I finished making the wheel and placing a paper fastener in the center, and I taped it to the gift. Instant bow.

Clubs

This is an area where likes attract, and you can develop an ongoing program. With just a few dollars for a camera, you can form a camera club or as I called ours—my Shutterbug Club. From this club, you can cover topics such as the use of a camera, lighting, portraits, building structure, landscape, and animals. At one of my classes, we took pictures of church doors. On the outing, we discussed color and design. Did the structure remind you of the coliseums of Rome or of some Greek structure you have seen in the past? I gave them new words like *Gothic* and *Roman architecture*. We developed the pictures and then discussed the positioning of the subject and how we could have improved the shot. We then followed up with designing a photo page in our album.

A club gives your client a sense of belonging to a special group. Let's face it, we all belong to groups, whether it is a church group or a service organization—they are a part of what make us who we are.

One of the important parts in a club is that each member gives some input, and that one or two people do not dominate the group. You may want to use the roundtable style where each person gets a chance to show and tell about their work.

Remember not to criticize their work and encourage positive facts to the group.

Music Appreciation

Everyone enjoys some type of music. The most important thing to remember is that the music you play for your client should be their choice, not yours. I am not saying that you can't play a certain type of music for a theme or celebration.

I remember many years ago that I attended a class on music appreciation, and how the instruction presented the class really made you think. When the class started, the instructor played a soft lullaby. After a few minutes, the instructor asked us how the music made us feel. He then put on a country tune, the volume a little louder. He played it for a few minutes and asked us once again to write down how the music made us feel. The last bit of music was "Stars and Stripes Forever," and this he played loud. The instructor asked us to write what we saw the other members doing. As you can guess, everyone agreed that the soft music made us feel one way, and the march made us feel another. In a matter of a few minutes, he changed how we felt by just changing the type and the volume of the music we were listening to.

In better restaurants, you often hear soft music, or they will have a piano player. At a Chinese restaurant, you would hear music of an Oriental flavor from the Far East. Both types of music will do the same thing, and that is to set the mood. When we hear "Hail to the Chief," we know we will see the president; and when at a wedding, when the "Wedding March" starts, we know to stand as the bride will be presented soon. Music is such an important part of our lives, and you should incorporate some when planning your activity calendar.

Many other activities can be designed around music. You could get a volunteer from your community or have another client play for you. You can have a sing-along or encourage a solo. You can make instruments and then put on a program. Creative activities could be to form a chorus or a rhythm band. Some clients will participate, and others may choose just to listen. Some music will become a form of exercise like a good old-fashioned square dance or Lindy, and other music may awaken emotions of the past. All the activities you plan will be centered on the population you serve. What is appropriate for their age? What time would be best to have this activity? Once you complete your assessment of the client, you will better understand what type of music you should plan. Each time you have a musical activity, make a mental note of what should stay the same and what should be changed.

Encourage the clients to share their thoughts, and if you have a volunteer guest, don't forget the thank-you note.

Attracting Birds

Watching and listening to our fine-feathered friends can give hours of enjoyment. How to get them to come to your yard is a simple task. Meet their needs of food, water, and shelter; and you will attract many different types of birds. It may be very rewarding to keep a journal, listing the birds that visit your feeder. Start by identification—what time of the day it visits the feeder and if you could tell if it was a male or female. List the colors of the bird and the number of birds you see. You may want to draw a picture or take a picture of them.

You can write your state college for information as to what to feed and what kind of birds are in your area. You can get more information at your public library. Some birds sing—they are noted as songbirds—others make a squawking sound. Remember that the sounds have meanings for other birds. Some sounds are for courting and others for warnings. Some may be telling location or may be indications of hunger. Whatever kind of bird-watching—making feeders, feeding, or drawing—you can plan many activities.

A simple platform feeder is just a piece of three-fourths plywood cut into twelve by twelve inches. Drill a few holes in the bottom to release any water. You may attach one-inch strips along the edges to hold the seed back.

Suet feeders attract birds too. We enjoy watching the woodpeckers come into ours. You can buy cakes at your local Agway or Wal-Mart, or you can add another activity in rendering down beef fat. For this project, you will have to cut beef fat into small pieces and run it through a grinder. (I found it already ground at my local supermarket.) Heat in a heavy skillet and cook until the suet congeals. Then let it cool completely and cook a second time. The suet should melt down. Pour into sandwich-size plastic containers and refrigerate until solid. Keep refrigerated until you're ready to set it out. I placed our suet in a (recycled) onion bag. When you have rendered down the fat the second time, you can add other ingredients like seeds, raisins, cornmeal, or peanut butter. Just add one-half cup of your choice to each cup of fat.

Writing

A piece of paper, a pen, and some imagination, and you have an activity. Writing is a record of your spoken or words of thought put down on paper. You can make someone laugh or cry in the sharing of your words. If you take to a pen for an activity, you will arouse a vision or evoke a feeling. Whether you write a short story, a bit of poetry, a card, or letter to a friend, this activity does not cost much. In fact, the therapeutic value far exceeds the cost. When I was working, I would gather four or five clients, and we would write a letter to servicemen. It was during Operation Desert Storm, and we wanted to help in some small way. We would sit down, and each person would write a few lines. One of my clients who did not like to participate in activities joined in because he was concerned about the war. This opened a door for me, and I looked for information, books, and news items to share with him. We enjoyed reading the letters we would receive from our servicemen. From time to time, we would talk to one of them on the phone. When our town had a parade, my client marched holding our special hero's picture. So you can see that our act of kindness became much more to the clients. We were not writing for publication, but we were cheering up a friend. We also sent newspaper clippings, funny stories, and our prayers. I may be retired now, but I still write the clients I cared for.

When you plan this type of activity, you must listen. I have learned a lot about my clients and their families over the years; and it is very important that you practice confidentiality and never be judgmental.

Keeping in touch with family is important to your client. Though far away, they still share that feeling of belonging. Encourage your client to write and read because this will offer another avenue for you to better understand them.

Seed Art

This is one of those projects I saw my mother do when I was a teenager. Mom's design was a wall plaque of a rooster. The base of the project was a piece of plywood cut from a drawing of a rooster. She marked off each section that would be a different seed. She had an assortment of large and small seeds and glued the seeds in each section. She gave the finished work a few coats of acrylic paint spray, and it was lovely. This is a basic skill that you can use to make a flower on a card, a photo frame, a wall plaque, and so much more. For our project, we bought a $1 wooden frame at a yard sale. We bought a mixed blend of birdseed at our local Agway. Look for blends with large and small seeds. Now, cover a section of the frame with glue and pour on the seed. Do this over a pan or box to catch falling seeds. When you have completed the frame, set it aside and let it dry. After the glue has dried completely, you can paint it any color you like. I used a gold spray just following the instructions on the can and working in a well-ventilated area. If you are going to brush on paint, do it very gently so you don't pull off the seeds. Let the paint dry and give it a second coat if necessary. If you are a patient person, you could position the seeds to form a design on the frame, and using a tweezers, dip each seed the glue, and then position it to form a unique design. This will take a long time, but your finished work will be a one-of-a-kind conversation piece. My mother's rooster plaque proudly hung in our kitchen for years, and many visitors were amazed when they learned that she made it from seeds.

Postcards

For this project, you will need one four-by-six inch file card, one four by photo of your client's choice, and a roll of double-sided tape. Draw a line to divide your card for the written message and a portion for the stamp and address, about three and one-half inches from the left edge of the card. You will write your message, jot down the address, and apply the stamp before you tape the photo on the other side of the card. Now turn your card over and apply double-sided tape around the edges of the card. For the last part, you will place your photo back to the taped side of file card. Press gently to make sure they are bonded.

Music Appreciation

Create an interest in different types of music. Play a marching tape and ask the client how the music makes them feel. Encourage physical involvement by clapping your hands or tapping your feet. You may wish to overlap activities by giving each client a marker and a piece of paper to draw what they feel. Listen to the music and see if marks show a rhythm. Remember to display the artwork. Exercise to music, dance, or just play soft music when a meal is being served. Have a musician come in and play the music they like and encourage them to sing or play instruments. If you have a client that can play an instrument, encourage them to participate. Form a chorus and have a hymn singing hour on Sunday afternoon. Take it outside when the weather is good. Be creative when it comes to music and name that tune.

Pasta for Use

Did you ever go to the supermarket and look at all the different types of pasta there? Well, I was looking at the small alphabets and thought they could be used on tags for gifts. And why not color them with a marker? Then I looked at the small pasta and noticed a variety of shapes. So why not put a border of pasta around your tag and color that too? Now my wheels are clicking. How about gluing pasta on a photo frame and painting the frame brown to give a carved-wood effect? How about a wall plaque? Draw a design on a piece of wood and fill in different areas with different-sized pasta. Paint the areas with different colors. You will have a one-of-a-kind piece of artwork. You can get small wooden cutouts at craft stores for Christmas ornaments. Why not make your ornaments with a bit of texture? Buy a few different types of pasta and keep them in glass jars—this will keep your pasta clean and avoid the company of furry little friends. If the background will be the same color as the pasta, you can paint everything at once. If your background is different, you can paint the pasta, let it dry, and then glue it to the painted background.

Wrapping Paper Art

Looking for a source of white paper (check Crayola banner paper). It is large enough for a banner, or you can cut it to make wrapping paper. For this project, you will use two pencils of contrasting colors. Place the pencils side by side and tape them together. Now, they should draw a double line spaced about one-fourth inch apart (you could use two pencils of the same color.) We are going to make a birthday wrapping paper, so let's write the words randomly all over the paper. If you know the person's name, you could also write that. Other methods of decorating the paper: use stickers, markers, paint, glue magazine pictures, stencil, or even finger paint to create interesting one-of-a-kind gift wrap. Don't forget to make a matching tag from a piece of card stock.

Door Stops

Know someone who is a bricklayer? Don't be shy. Ask for some used or damaged bricks to use for this project. Be sure the brick is clean and free from dust; just have your client clean them off with a sturdy brush. Give the brick a coat or two of paint and decorate by painting a second color with a sponge for contrast. If your client can use a stencil or draw their own picture, they could do that as well. Our clients used a stencil of a goose, and every time I see one of the bricks, I laugh because they have been around for years.

Mobiles

Mobiles are another craft that can change with the monthly theme or as a seasonal focal point. One time, when I was in Maine with a client, we went to a restaurant, and I saw one made of old silverware. It made a soft sound in the dining room and was a neat conversation piece. Ask your maintenance department to keep you in mind when they pull out that old copper plumbing or just ask your friendly plumber for five pieces in different lengths. Drill a hole about one-half inch from the edge. Sand the rough spots for safety. Other materials needed are a clapper and a circle of wood to hold your hanging pipes. I didn't have wood, so I used a canning ring to hang my pipes from. I just drilled five evenly spaced holes to hold the fishing line and pipe, and the lid became the clapper, hanging down through the center to tap the pipes in the wind. I just painted it black on both sides. Oh, I also painted the ring black too.

Pincushion

Recycle a tuna fish can. Wash and remove the label from a tuna fish can and paint the can. When the paint has dried, place one old knee-high nylon stocking in the bottom of the can and cover with a piece of batting cut to fit on top. Take a nice decorative piece of material and cover the cotton batting. You can glue everything by running some hot glue around the inner rim of the can. You could finish it off with a piece of lace or ribbon to cover the rim or just hot glue some beads around the edge. Be creative with what you have.

Wreaths

Wreaths can be placed on the door or on a wall as art. You can buy bear wreaths at craft stores or thrift shops. We made roses from photocopies of music sheets. We added five gold angel ornaments and a big red bow too. For the rose, take a paper rose apart, and you will see the pattern you will need. Lay the pattern on a piece of music paper and trace out your pattern. Cut out as many as you need to complete your rose. Run a wire around the base to attach the rose to your wreath. Add your own final decorations, bow, and hanger for the back; and you have a great gift for your volunteer musician.

Season's Greetings

Cut a band of white paper to fit around your favorite candy bar. We used a Hershey's bar because it has a nice flat surface. Now just decorate the wrapper to make it special. We made ours for Christmas, so we wrote Season's Greetings, You Sweet Thing! But you could write a special note like Happy Birthday; Happy Valentine's Day, Sweetie; or Happy New Year. You can color the wrapper or place stickers on it too. Once your work of art is complete, place the wrapper around your candy bar and place a piece of clear tape to hold it in place.

A Photo Puzzle

For this project, you will need one eight-by-ten inch photo, one eight-by-ten inch copy of a photo, and some glue. You will glue the photo to the piece of cardboard. Let the board dry completely. Turn the board over and draw one-inch lines vertically and horizontally. Cut on the lines for form your one-inch squares. Mix up the pieces, turn them over, and put your personal puzzle together. Just for fun, send the pieces to a family or friend to put together.

Tissue Box Cover

For the pattern, open your favorite brand of tissue box. Lay it flat on a piece of white poster paper. Trace around your pattern with a pencil and cut it out. Now find the section that would be the bottom and cut it off. You don't need it because this is going to be the opening to place over your tissue box. Don't forget to cut out the hole where the tissues come out of. Reassemble your tissue box and set it aside. Now is the time to decorate your cover. We made our covers for Father's Day and wrote Number 1 Dad on the top, and the clients gave them to their fathers to keep in their cars. You could make this a seasonal decoration by covering the white cutout with wrapping paper or make it personal by adding a person's name in bold letters. When you have completed your masterpiece, you will have to glue your project together just like your master box. I think this project sounds harder than it really is.

Wreath Centerpiece

Wreaths can be placed on your front door, put on a wall for art, or placed on your table as a centerpiece. You can change the decorations on the wreath to match a special holiday or event. Pinecones, walnut shells, twigs—all can be used as fillers. Add some Christmas ornaments or artificial flowers for additional interest. You may glue on some permanent pieces of decoration in place and just tuck in those that you will be changing.

Word Games

Many years ago, I used to work in a factory, and the way it was set up was that machine operators sat facing each other so they could talk as they worked. Well, I used to sit across from a wonderful lady who enjoyed playing games as we worked. Little did I know that twenty years later, I would use these skills to plan activities for my clients. All you have to do is make a list of things—let's say cars. Start with the letter *A* and name a car; then, I would name a car using the letter *B*, and then we would go back to her for the letter *C*. We really got quite competitive some days. You can name the states, birds, flowers, or types of ice cream.

Bible Study

Each Sunday, church bulletins take a passage from the Bible and have a written story for you to read. I collected several of the bulletins and formed a Bible study group. We would read the passage and then discuss the meaning. Check with your local pastors for information and see if the church has a Bible study program.

Flower Press

Many years ago, I wanted to make a flower press so that I could make my own cards for a special occasion. For this, I had a friend cut two pieces of plywood into twelve by twelve inches, and I had a hole five-sixteenth of an inch drilled neatly in each corner about one-half inch from the edge. I sanded the edges and the drilled hole spaces nice and smooth. I bought four six-inch carriage bolts, four wing nuts, and eight washers. I made the inserts by cutting six pieces of cardboard ten-by-ten inches and covered the cardboard with white construction paper. I thought the construction would absorb the moisture from the plants. Now you think that the project, once put together, is over. Well, not for me. I took out a wood-burning tool and went to work. I wrote the word Flower and burned in a large rose. I then painted the leaves green and the rose red and let the paint dry. For my last step, I applied five coats of polyurethane. I brought the press to work, and we enjoyed pressing flowers and making cards. This is one project that will last for years.

That's a Roma

To practice diversity, you may wish to celebrate another nationality. If you have staffs from another country, encourage them to help design a program or programs leading up a big celebration. Think about the culture and what is unique about them. Foods and dancing could be activities. Regional foods usually are based on foods grown in that area. Check at your local library for books and tapes too.

Bookmarker Thong

When I first saw these at Borders, I laughed. Then I started looking at them, and the idea was a good one. So I thought why not make an activity using ribbon and maybe charms or buttons. Well, this is what you will need: two pieces of two-by-one inch card stock, a piece of twelve-by-three-fourths inch ribbon, six small buttons, and glue. You will glue the card stock to the ends of the ribbon, and then glue the buttons on the card stock. Let it dry completely. We were lucky when we did this activity because we used recycled ribbon and buttons. When it comes to recycling, you should try to do it every day in some way.

Party Hats

When I was a kid, we made party hats from recycled newspaper or brown shopping bags. You could use those materials or make them from paper plates, tissue paper, and poster paper or even wallpaper. For our project, we cut a band into five by twenty-four inches from poster paper. We cut one top edge in a sawtooth pattern and decorate the band with markers. We then glued some gems four inches apart for more interest. For the ladies, you may want to glue some feathers around the edge or mix in some flowers and ribbon.

Newsletter

This could be fun and also an avenue to pass information to family and friends. Articles should be positive, and information should be correct. It could be a time to project upcoming events or to share goals set for the future. Clients could have a column, take part in corresponding, or help in the mailing.

Straw Hat Art

Looking at the hat, we see two pieces—the brim and the head or crown. We think of the crown as the face and will position the eyes, nose, and mouth in their proper place. We could cut a second smaller hat and position it on the top of the crown. You could use raffia or yarn for hair and place ears for added interest. This is what I call the "bones" of the project. At Easter, we made a rabbit. We painted a sixteen-inch white straw hat and cut a twelve-inch hat in one-half to put on the top of the head. We made ears by cutting pink colored paper for the center and white ones for the outer part. We applied cotton to the edge of the white area on the ear too. I made two teeth from craft foam, and we used black chenille to make the whiskers. We placed eyelashes and craft eyes to complete our face. We added a large pink bow below the face, and our project was complete.

Visit a Local Newspaper

For this community interaction project, we arranged a tour of one of our local newspaper shops. We were guided through each step and met people working at different stations. On our trip, the reporter wrote a headline that we had saved the day in large letters. They showed us how the master copy was made and then the steps in using the printing machine. We all went home with a copy of the special newspaper.

Visit the Local Jail

Our visit to the local jail not only was a trip, but it became a history lesson as well. We visited the old jail, which was open to the public for tours now. The past mayor and a friend of mine for many years were the tour guide. We were given the royal visitors' tour, and we hit it just right to meet the current sheriff. He discussed the old jail and how it was outdated, and he told us about the new jail. He gave us an invitation to visit that building too.

Airport

Sometimes, you will have clients that travel, and then you may have a client who has never been to an airport. A trip to the airport has changed since 9/11, and you may wish to find a smaller local airfield. We took a trip to a small airport, which had a diner where the clients could sit, eat lunch, and watch planes take off and land. I found that this was a better event for my clients. Always keep in mind that your activity should not cause stress to the client or yourself. I felt going to an airport with five people could be modified just by downsize of the airport.

Radio Station and Television Studio

You should make an appointment for your trip to the local station. You should explain who you are and inform them of your special needs. You may wish to keep the tour down to a certain time span like thirty minutes or one hour. Do your homework with regard to stairs, parking, and other services they have for your handicapped population. Our trip was to the local television station, and our clients knew everyone they met by name. The social interaction was like the people were our friends. I guess because you see them every day, you may feel like you know them. Don't forget to send a thank-you card or make a certification of appreciation.

Postcard Art

For this project, you will need a four-by-six photo, a four-by-six file card, a ruler, pen, and double-sided tape. If you look at the store-bought type of card, you will see a line dividing the message part and the address section, so place a line down the middle of your file card on the plain side. You will place your message on the left side portion of the card and your mailing address on the right side section. On the line side of the file card, run the tape as close to the edge as you can and tape all four edges. Now for the tricky part, lay the back side of your photo over the tape on the card and gently press down. You can make your own Christmas postcard by taking your client's picture in front of some pricey decorations at the mall or maybe building a snowman. After a client receives a gift, take a picture of the client with the gift, all smiles, check your background, and make a thank-you postcard. You could make invitations to a party by giving the date, time, place, and RSVP information too. Share with family and friends pictures of your client on day trips and doing a special activity. They say one picture can say a thousand words, so share your special time together.

Potpourri

When I was a child, we used to make a potpourri bundle to put in our underwear drawer. Nothing fancy, just a collection of pine needles placed in a cotton cloth bag about two by three inches when finished. You can make a scented pillow by collecting lavender flowers or rose petals and putting them in one of those cloth bags they use for favors at bridal showers, or you could sew your own. You will need two pieces of a thin material cut 2 ½ x 3 ½, a needle, and thread. Sew three sides of your pillow closed, and then place your flowers inside. If you like the smell of cinnamon, allspice, or clove, you could add a few tablespoons of that too. Sew the last side closed, and you have completed your pillow—or have you? If you use a plain white cotton bag for your project, you could add another personal touch by putting your name on the bag written with a fabric marker or sewing a charm or two to make a one-of-a-kind pillow. Why not make them as party favors? Your room will have a pleasant aroma, and your guests will have a keepsake gift as well.

Drawing

Give a small child a crayon, and he will draw on a piece of paper or maybe the wall. The need to draw is something that it seems we may inherit. I think way back, the caveman drew on the walls of his cave, and I don't know why. It seems it is just something we do. So knowing this is an enjoyable experience for most people, put it on your activity calendar at least once a month. Don't worry if the drawings aren't da Vinci's or Michelangelo's because I bet their first drawings weren't that great too. Remember you are not drawing for a living, you are drawing for fun.

What's that you say? You can't draw well? Then trace a picture. After you trace the picture's outline, you can duplicate it for your file and refine the image. For our project, we traced a teacup in the lower right corner of our paper. Then we decorated the teacup with stickers of hearts. We folded the paper in half and then in half again so that the picture would be on the front of the card. We wrote a personal note inside, and it made a lovely card. Go one step further, and with a utility knife, make a cut on the rim of the cup large enough to slide in a tea bag, and you will have a card with an aroma.

Don't let their talents be hindered by inferior tools. I'm not saying buy professional equipment, but don't waste your money either. Buying drawing supplies will need your attention and thought about what you are drawing. You should have a set of colored pencils too. You will also need some drawing paper. If it is a work of art you wish to save for all time, you will need an acid-free paper. For most of my projects, I use a simple beginner's sketchbook—the eight-by-ten size.

Crayons

Crayons may be your choice; they are not just for kids anymore. The medium is important, but what is being colored should always be age appropriate.

Water Colors

This is a difficult medium. Controlling the amount of water is a science, which I'll admit I never conquered. Here is where you might say that less is best. You don't want your colors running into each other, do you? Your activity will also need a place to dry. When you are working with watercolors, you should put down some paper to absorb excess water. When finished, you can just toss everything in the trash, and everyone should take part in cleaning up. Keeping brushes clean is a must, so make sure they are clean and dry before you put them away.

Charcoal

This is a messy form of art. Your hands are going to get dirty. When we learn to draw, part of our hand is always resting on the paper for stability. Well, you can't do that with charcoal. You need to keep your hand off the paper. I like to use pastel colors and black construction paper. You can encourage blending with the use of a finger or a piece of tissue.

Pens

No permanent markers. We had a rule—no permanent markers at all, and I really don't think I have to explain why. There are several types of pens, and over the years, I guess I tried them all. You should have a box or two in your supplies.

Papier-Mâché Mask

When making the paste to hold the papier-mâché, mix equal parts of water and flour. You could also use liquid starch and cold water again in equal parts. For your project, you will tear strips of newspaper and dip the paper into the mixture. You will then apply it to a form of chicken wire, cardboard, or even a balloon. You will need to let each coat dry overnight. You could make masks by covering a large balloon—say as big as your head. Apply four or five layers, let each dry. You should pop the balloon with a pin and then cut the finished piece in half. You will need to paint your "face" and apply facial features. You could apply yarn on the top for hair. Dress it up with glasses and be creative—remember, it's one of a kind.

You will need to paper punch two holes for the ribbon so you can tie it behind your head. You could make a form, let's say an animal, and cover it with papier-mâché. Paint it and decorate it. This would be a great project if you were in a parade.

The first fact is the recipe, and then the most important is your imagination.

Cinnamon / Applesauce Dough

Mix equal parts of cinnamon and applesauce to form dough.
This is a dough that should be listed under aromatherapy. This is a bit messy, but it is worth it. This project should air-dry for a couple of days. If you need to place a hole in it for hanging, you need to do it before drying.

Once you form your dough, roll it out just like you would cookie dough. In fact, you now can use a cookie cutter and cut out a shape.

I did this with my clients, and we used a heart-shape cutter. We used a pencil to punch a hole in the top (before drying) and ran a red ribbon for a hanger after it was dry. We gave them out on Valentine's Day. This is one project where the heart smelled great for months.
You could also shape this dough and add other elements to make it personal.

Flour and Salt Dough

This, again, is one of those recipes that come from items found in the kitchen. One important note here: if you are sensitive to salt, wear thin rubber gloves. It is recommended that everyone using this recipe wash their hands well after the project is over. For the dough, mix two cups of flour, one cup of salt, and enough water to make a dough. We made a batch of dough and rolled it into small balls. We ran a wire through the bead and baked it for one and a half hours at three hundred degrees. We removed them from the oven and let them cool. For the next part of the project, we painted the beads. We removed the wire and used some dental floss to join the beads. We tied a knot at the end, and we had a one-of-a-kind work of art. Don't forget to make the strand long enough that when it is tied, you can fit it over your head.

This can be a seasonal project—red, white, and blue beads for June, July, and September respectively.
Orange and black for Halloween while red and green for Christmas.

Potato Stamping

When I was growing up, we didn't have a lot of money, so Mom made do with things around the house, and the potato stamp was one of those crafts.

Materials:

> One large potato
> One cookie cutter
> Sharp paring knife
> Card stock
> Paint or ink

Wash potato and dry with paper towel; cut potato in half lengthwise. Insert cookie cutter about one-half inch. Now with the paring knife, cut off excess potato around the cookie cutter about one-half inch. Remove cookie cutter and pat dry potato with paper towel. Dip cut-cookie pattern on the potato into paint, blot off excess paint, and press on to paper. Lift potato stamp straight up as not to smudge the paint. You should have your cookie design on the paper.

This is a great project to design wrapping paper, bookmarkers, or even a photo frame if the cutter is small enough.

Horticulture
Square-Foot Gardening

Step one design. Each plot is four-by-four feet and is divided into 1 sixteen-by-one feet sections. Each plot has an aisle around it three feet wide. This may sound like a lot, but when your garden starts to grow, the space will become smaller.

What to plant. Vegetables or flowers—well, maybe both.
Tomato plants do well when planted next to marigolds because marigolds keep some of the garden pests away.

Remember to start small.

C	L	T	M
C	L	T	M
C	L	T	M
C	L	T	M

C: cucumbers
L: lettuce
T: tomato
M: marigolds

Therapeutic values: education, cooperation, and patience.

Keeping the Faith

Passover is an important Jewish holiday, so we have a discussion and serve some traditional foods. As you are working with clients, ask them to tell you why this holiday is important to them, and how they celebrated it in the past. See if there are family traditions you can include in your activity. Some music, a reading from the Bible, or a special blessing would be nice too.

Potato Latkes

Ten medium potatoes
One medium onions
Two large eggs
One-fourth cup unbleached all purpose flour, breadcrumbs, or matzo meal
Salt and pepper to taste
Vegetable oil for frying

Grate potatoes and onion. Add eggs and seasoning. Place small amount of oil on a griddle then drop one-fourth cup of mixture on the pan and fry on both sides till golden brown and fork-tender. Serve with applesauce or sour cream.

You can keep potato cakes warm in oven set at two hundred degrees till ready to serve.

For your documentation, the therapeutic value is keeping one's faith through traditional foods and cooking skills. Remember safety in the kitchen.

Animal Shelter

This will be a community interaction project and cooking class project too. The staff will call the shelter to discuss their wants and needs and see how our community project will help. Check the day and time to bring supplies and gifts to the shelter.

Cooking project: Clients will make microwave morsels to present as a gift.

Microwave Morsels

Two chicken bouillon cubes
One cup of boiling water
Two cups of whole wheat flour
One-half cup of stone-ground cornmeal
One and one-half cups of powdered skim milk
One cup of quick-cooking rolled oats
One-half cup of vegetable oil
Two beaten eggs

Dissolve bouillon cubes in water and set aside. In a large mixing bowl, combine dry ingredients. Mix well and then add oil, eggs, and bouillon immersed in water to mix. Knead dough on floured surface four to five millimeters. Roll dough to one-half inch thickness. Cut with dog biscuit cutter and place on a microproof dish. Microwave it for five minutes, turn and microwave five more minutes, turn again and microwave for another five minutes.

Cool on a rack and store in sealed plastic bags in the refrigerator.

For your documentation, the activity provides creative expression and community interaction.

Keepsake Album

For this project, you will need two pieces of cardboard, three beads, heavy-duty string, glue, paper for filler, and paper to decorate the covers.

Cut the cardboard one inch larger than your filler paper. Have clients decorate the cover page. Have markers, pencils, crayons, cutout pictures from magazines or photos—this is a time to be creative.

Run tape around the edges of the book. I used a two-inch duct tape because of its durability, but you can use masking tape or whatever is available. This will give the cover a nice finished edge. You will cover most of the tape when you put down the cover page. The cover page should be the same size as the cardboard. You can decorate both the front and back.

You will have to punch holes in the cover to match the holes in the paper. Then insert the beads and run the string through the beads to secure. Note that you may want to make a sample first.

For your documentation, the activity provides, creative expression, and memory stimulation.

Fire Prevention Week

Fire prevention is an important part of everyone's life, and it can be an interesting activity. Start with the historical background of why we have Fire Prevention Week and why the dates are important. Read about the Great Chicago Fire of 1871. Most of the city was destroyed, and 250 people died.

Contact your local fire department for materials and events.

Evacuation: what is your plan?

Invite your fire chief to lunch and make a donation to the fire department.

Have a fire drill and discuss how it went, how it could be improved, and think of areas where fires start.

What should you do if your clothes catch on fire? Stop, drop, and roll.

Fire Prevention Week is time set aside, but prevention is an everyday concern.

Bits and Pieces

Range of motion. When it hurts, *stop*. You do not know each person's range of motion. You could cause damage by extending past the point of discomfort. Remember, you are in charge of the client's safety while in your care. You have to be aware of areas where they could get hurt, and you need to know what to do in the event of an injury. You need to protect the client and yourself. In the event that a client is injured while in your care, get help and document, document, document. You need to evaluate why it happened and a course of action to prevent this from happening again. Believe me when I say that to have a client injured while in your care can be life-changing to both of you.

Community connection. It is important that your client be a part of the community, and if possible, join a club or do some volunteer service. When you complete your client assessment, you may find that they are in a service organization. If not, help them to become a member or do some volunteer service. It is important for each person's social skills and that we feel needed or a have connection to something larger. You will see that the client maintains or improves their social skills and has a sense of self-worth.

Religious belief. Most people have a religious belief, and within a religion, people tend to have a sense of self-belief. Sometimes, these variables occur because of family tradition or the country they came from. Very often, you will find that within a church, people have opposing ideas. Now when it comes to your client, they will have their own belief as well. You'll need to put your beliefs in check, be neutral, and meet their need to maintain their individuality. You may want to learn as much as you can about their religion because you can plan many activities to celebrate their faith. I learned how to make challah bread to serve on the Sabbath for a client of Jewish faith. We enjoyed making the bread, and now I make the bread on special holidays for my family too.

Diversity. Webster's Dictionary says it is a variety of something such as opinion, color, style, or ethnic variety, as well as socioeconomic and gender variety in a group, society, or institution. It seems we are becoming a country with global diversification (I just made up that word). What I am trying to say is that we are made up of many different ethnic and cultural groups, and you may have a client that at first, you don't understand. Some customs practiced may be very foreign to your ideas. All I can say here is learn to know your client, and don't be judgmental. I am not saying you have to give up your beliefs, but it is your job to respect you client's wishes. If, for some religious reasons, you cannot participate in the activity and you can get someone else to take it, please do so. This is an area of mutual respect. I should say here that you should know the staff you are working with and try to avoid this problem. Don't plan an activity you know a coworker would be uncomfortable doing. Speaking of coworkers, know their strengths and weakness too. Know their talents and what they enjoy doing with the client. For you and your part, all I can say is don't hog all the good activities and remember you are part of a team. A good supervisor will monitor this and maybe set up some house rules. I think if a person goes through all the trouble of designing an outing or activity, they should have first choice on whether they want to do it. Please encourage team participation. The client will benefit with this approach.

I have collected over the past twenty years the bits and pieces of time. I have tested and perfected the activities—keeping in mind the wants, needs, and wishes of my clients.

I hope that in sharing these facts and lessons, you are inspired to present activities that will enrich the moments you spend with your clients because that is what life is—just a collection of moments in time.

May God bless you and your work,

Margaret Martone

www.ingramcontent.com/pod-product-compliance
Lightning Source LLC
Chambersburg PA
CBHW031304280526
45784CB00004B/1989